CERTIFICATE OF INCORPORATION

AND

CONSTITUTION AND BY-LAWS

OF THE

BUFFALO HISTORICAL SOCIETY

AS AMENDED JANUARY 12, 1867.

TO WHICH IS ADDED

A LIST OF THE OFFICERS, STANDING COMMITTEES, AND MEMBERS.

INCORPORATED JANUARY, 1863.

BUFFALO:
THOMAS, HOWARD & JOHNSON.
FRANKLIN PRINTING HOUSE.
1868.

CERTIFICATE OF INCORPORATION

AND

CONSTITUTION AND BY-LAWS

OF THE

BUFFALO HISTORICAL SOCIETY

AS AMENDED JANUARY 12, 1867.

TO WHICH IS ADDED

A LIST OF THE OFFICERS, STANDING COMMITTEES, AND MEMBERS.

INCORPORATED JANUARY, 1863.

BUFFALO:
THOMAS, HOWARD & JOHNSON.
FRANKLIN PRINTING HOUSE.
1868.

CERTIFICATE OF INCORPORATION.

We, the undersigned citizens and residents of the City of Buffalo, within the State of New York, of the full age of twenty-one years and upwards, and citizens of the United States, do, pursuant to the statute in such case made and provided, hereby associate ourselves together, and form a Corporation, or Society, for Historical purposes.

The name or title by which such Society or Corporation shall be known in law, is "The Buffalo Historical Society." The particular business and object of such Society and its general design is, to discover, procure, and preserve whatever may relate to the History of Western New York, and the City of Buffalo in particular, and likewise aim to gather statistics of the commerce, manufactures, and business of the Lake region, and those portions of the West that are intimately connected with the interests of Buffalo.

The Officers of such Society shall be a President, a Vice President, a Recording Secretary, and a Corresponding Secretary and Librarian, Treassurer, and nine Councillors, who, together, shall constitute the Board of Managers of said Society. The number of Managers of said Society, as aforesaid, shall be fourteen, and their names for the first year of its existence, are as follows:

MILLARD FILLMORE, *President.*
LEWIS F. ALLEN, *Vice President.*
CHARLES D. NORTON, *Recording Secretary.*
GUY H. SALISBURY, *Cor. Sec'y and Librarian.*
OLIVER G. STEELE, *Treasurer.*

COUNCILLORS.

George R. Babcock,
William Dorsheimer,
William Shelton,
Walter Clarke,
Orsamus H. Marshall,
Henry W. Rogers,
Nathan K. Hall,
George W. Clinton,
George W. Hosmer.

The principal office and place of business of such Society, shall be located at said City of Buffalo, in the County of Erie.

We, the undersigned members, officers, and managers of such Society, do hereby certify the matters above stated, to the end that we, our associates and successors, may, pursuant to the statute of the State aforesaid, in such case made and provided, be a body politic and corporate, by the name above stated, and in witness whereof, we have severally hereunto subscribed our names, the thirty-first day of December, 1862.

G. W. CLINTON,
ASHER P. NICHOLS,
WM. DORSHEIMER,
OLIVER G. STEELE,
HENRY W. ROGERS,

{ Stamp. 10 cents. }

MILLARD FILLMORE,
LEWIS F. ALLEN,
GUY H. SALISBURY,
W. A. BIRD,
GEO. R. BABCOCK,
O. H. MARSHALL,
JOHN B. SKINNER,
HENRY DAW.

COUNTY OF ERIE, } ss.
CITY OF BUFFALO, }

On this sixth day of January, 1863, personally appeared before me, George W. Clinton, Asher P. Nichols, William Dorsheimer, Millard Fillmore, Lewis F. Allen, Guy H. Salisbury, Oliver G. Steele, William A. Bird, Henry W. Rogers, George R. Babcock, Orsamus H. Marshall, John B. Skinner, and Henry Daw, severally known to me to be the persons described in, and who executed the above instrument, and they severally acknowledged the execution of the same.

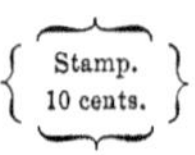

M. P. FILLMORE,
Commissioner of Deeds
For the City of Buffalo.

The undersigned, one of the Justices of the Supreme Court for the Eighth Judicial District of the State of New York, hereby consents to, and approves of the filing of the annexed certificate, for the incorporation of the Buffalo Historical Society.

Dated January 8, 1863. R. P. MARVIN.

Filed in the office of the Secretary of State, of the State of New York, and in the office of the Clerk of the County of Erie, January 10, 1863.

CONSTITUTION.

1. This Society shall be called "THE BUFFALO HISTORICAL SOCIETY."

2. The general object of the Society shall be, to discover, procure and preserve whatever may relate to the history of Western New York in general, and the city of Buffalo in particular, and to gather statistics of the commerce, manufactures and business of the lake region, and those portions of the West that are intimately connected with the business of Buffalo.

3. The Society shall consist of resident, corresponding and honorary members, who shall be elected by a majority of ballots; and of life members, as hereinafter provided. Resident members shall consist of persons residing in the city of Buffalo or County of Erie; corresponding and honorary members, of persons residing elsewhere.

4. The officers of the Society shall consist of a President, a Vice President, a Recording Secretary, a Corresponding Secretary and Librarian, a Treasurer, and nine Councillors, who shall be elected annually, on the second Tuesday of January in each year, by a majority of ballots, and who shall constitute the Board of Managers of the Society.

5. None but resident and life members shall be eligible to office or qualified to vote.

6. Resident members shall pay an admission fee of five dollars, and also an annual due of five dollars, which shall be paid on or before the first day of November in each calendar year, after that

in which they shall have been elected. The election of a resident member shall confer no privilege of membership, until his admission fee shall be paid. The payment of the annual dues shall be a condition of continued membership, and any member neglecting to pay his annual due before the first day of January next after it becomes payable, shall thereby forfeit all his privileges of membership.

7. The payment of fifty dollars, at one time, for that purpose, shall constitute a life member, exempt from all annual dues.

8. The Society shall meet monthly, on the second Tuesday in every month. The President, or, in his absence, the Vice President, or either of the Secretaries, may direct the call of a special meeting in such manner as the By-Laws shall provide.

9. Those members who shall attend at any meeting of the Society, shall constitute a quorum for the transaction of business.

10. All officers shall continue in office until their successors are elected or appointed. Their duties, when not herein defined, may be prescribed by the By-Laws. All vacancies in office may be filled for the unexpired term, at any regular meeting of the Society.

11. This Constitution may be amended from time to time by a majority vote of the members present at a regular meeting, provided notice of the proposed amendments be given at least four weeks previous to a final vote thereon.

BY-LAWS.

1. The meetings of this Society shall be held at the rooms of the Society, or at such other place as the President may appoint, and at such hour as shall be designated by the Secretary in the notice of the meeting.

2. The Recording or Corresponding Secretary shall give notice of each meeting, by previous publication of the same in one or more of the daily papers of the city.

3. Any meeting may be adjourned to such time as a majority of the members present shall determine.

4. The President shall preside at all the meetings of the Society, regulate its proceedings, preserve order and decorum, and have a casting vote. He shall also be the Chairman of the Board of Managers.

5. The Vice President shall discharge all the duties of the President in case of his absence.

6. The Recording Secretary shall have the custody of the Constitution, By-Laws, and Records of the Society. He shall give due notice of all its meetings, and keep a record of the same. He shall be the Secretary of the Board of Managers, and keep a record of its proceedings.

7. The Corresponding Secretary shall have the custody of all letters and communications on the business of the Society, and shall read to the Society all communications received by him as such Secretary. He shall, under the direction of the Society, pre-

pare all communications to be addressed to others in the name of the Society, and keep true copies of the same.

8. The Librarian, under the direction of the Board of Managers, shall have the custody of the library and cabinet, including all manuscripts, papers, documents, coins and maps, and shall, under the direction of the Board of Managers, provide cases suitable for their preservation, and for convenient reference and inspection. He shall keep a record of all donations, and report the same from time to time to the Society.

9. The Treasurer shall receive and keep all securities and sums of money due and payable or belonging to the Society. He shall keep the funds of the Society on deposit, to his credit as such Treasurer, in some safe institution, to be approved by the Board of Managers, and shall pay all such sums as the Board of Managers shall direct, on the written order or warrant of the President. He shall keep a true account of his receipts and disbursements, and render an annual statement thereof, and oftener if called upon by the Society or the Board of Managers. He may be required to give security for the faithful discharge of his duties, in such sum and form as the Board of Managers shall direct.

10. It shall be the duty of the Board of Managers to control and manage the affairs and funds of the Society. They shall make annually, on the second Tuesday of January, a report to the Society of its acquisitions and transactions for the preceding year.

11. All books, maps, manuscripts, and other articles belonging to the Society, shall be plainly marked with the name of the Society, and numbered, and entered in a catalogue arranged for convenient reference.

12. No books, maps, charts, manuscripts, or copies thereof, or any other article belonging to the library or cabinet, shall be taken therefrom without the written permission of a majority of the Board of Managers.

13. Any of these By-Laws may be suspended in case of a temporary exigency, by the unanimous vote of a meeting duly organ-

ized. They may be amended from time to time by a majority vote of the members present at a regular meeting, provided notice of the proposed amendment be given at least four weeks previous to a final vote thereon.

14. Any member of this Society may be expelled by the affirmative vote of two-thirds of all the resident members present at a regular meeting, but no such vote shall be taken unless notice of the motion to expel shall have been given at a meeting held at least four weeks previous thereto.

15. On the second Tuesday of January in each year, there shall be an address delivered before the Society, by some person to be appointed by the Board of Managers.

16. At the meetings of the Society, and (so far as may be applicable) at the meetings of the Board of Managers, the following shall be the order of business:

1. Reading of the minutes of the last meeting.
2. Reports and communications from the Officers of the Society.
3. Reports from Committees.
4. Election of members.
5. Miscellaneous business.
6. Reading of Papers and delivery of Addresses.

17. As soon as convenient after the annual election of officers, the President shall appoint from the Board of Managers, the following Standing Committees, to consist of three members each, viz.:

1. On Finance.
2. On the Library.
3. On Papers and Property.
4. On Donations, Subscriptions and Collections.
5. On Publications.
6. On Membership.

18. The President shall be, *ex officio*, Chairman of the Committee on Finance; and it shall be the duty of such Committee to take the general charge and supervision of the books, accounts,

and reports of the Treasurer, and of the finances, receipts, and expenditures of the Society. It shall also be its duty to consider and recommend all suitable measures to increase the revenues of the Society, and promote economy in its expenditures. It shall examine and report upon all accounts and claims against the Society, and upon all propositions for the appropriation or expenditure of its funds, when such propositions have not been reported upon, or made, by some other Committee of the Board.

19. The Committee on the Library shall have the general charge and supervision of the Library, and of all propositions and measures in regard to its increase, use, and management; or in regard to the procurement, exchange, or other disposition of books, periodicals, and pamphlets, or their binding or preservation. They shall cause a full and perfect catalogue of the books, periodicals, and pamphlets, belonging to the same, to be made, and, from time to time, corrected, continued, and kept, in order to facilitate reference thereto, and secure proper accountability therefor.

20. The Committee on Papers and Property shall have the general charge and supervision of all the papers and other property of the Society which shall not be catalogued as a part of its Library, and thus placed in the special charge of the Committee on the Library Committee. It shall be its duty to cause a full and perfect list, or inventory, of the same to be made, continued, and kept; and to propose to the Board, and carry into execution, (after the approval of the Board of Managers has been obtained,) such measures as may be deemed expedient for the classification, arrangement, care, preservation, and security of such papers, or, for obtaining papers or articles of historical or local interest for preservation by the Society.

21. The Committee on Donations, Subscriptions and Collections, shall have the general supervision and charge of procuring donations to the Society, and subscriptions to its funds, or for any special object. It shall also have charge of the collection thereof, and of all debts, and annual or other dues, to which the Society may be entitled; and it shall be its duty to propose proper meas-

ures for procuring donations and subscriptions, and for the prompt collection of all such subscriptions, debts and dues.

22. The Committee on Publications shall have the charge and supervision of all publications made by the direction of the Society, and shall carefully examine all papers and other things directed to be published, in order to discover all errors and defects, and procure the correction and remedy thereof. It shall also be their duty to make, or cause to be made, for publication, such abstracts or abridgments of papers as may be required, unless some other Committee shall have been charged with that duty.

23. It shall be the duty of the Committee on Membership to consider and report upon all questions relating to membership, which may be referred for that purpose, and, as far as practicable, to induce all proper persons to become members of the Society.

24. As soon as convenient after the annual election of officers, the President shall appoint the following Committees, each to consist of three members of the Society, not Managers, viz.:

1. On the Increase of the Library.
2. On the Increase of Members.
3. On Donations and Subscriptions.
4. On Statistics.
5. On Portraits, Pictures, and Photographs.
6. On Local History.
7. On Indian Reminiscences, Memorials, and History.

25. It shall be the duty of the Committee on the Increase of the Library, to procure donations of books and pamphlets; to endeavor, by other means, to increase the Library, and to propose to the Board of Managers such measures for its increase, as may be deemed expedient.

26. It shall be the duty of the Committee on the Increase of Members, to take all proper measures to increase the number of life and resident members; of the Committee on Donations and Subscriptions, to endeavor to increase the funds and property of the Society, by donations and legacies, and otherwise; of the Com-

mittee on Statistics, to collect, digest, arrange, and put in suitable form for preservation and use, the statistics of the commerce, manufactures, and business of the City of Buffalo and the Lakes, and of those portions of the West which are intimately connected with the business of Buffalo; of the Committee on Portraits, Pictures, and Photographs, to obtain donations of portraits, pictures, and photographs, and especially of portraits in oil of early settlers and other citizens; of the Committee on Local History, to procure, digest, arrange, and put in proper order for preservation and use, materials for a history of the City of Buffalo, and of the several towns of the County of Erie; and of the Committee on Indian Reminiscences, Memorials and History, to discover, collect, and arrange in suitable form for preservation and use, whatever they can obtain relating to the habits, peculiarities, possessions, and history of the Indian Nations and Tribes, now, or formerly, occupying portions of this State.

27. All reports of Standing Committees shall be in writing, but they may report by resolution if they shall deem it expedient.

Officers of the Society.

1868.

HENRY W. ROGERS, *President.*

ALBERT T. CHESTER, D. D., *Vice President.*

WILLIAM C. BRYANT, *Recording Secretary.*

GEORGE S. ARMSTRONG, *Cor. Secretary and Librarian.*

OLIVER G. STEELE, *Treasurer.*

Councillors.

WILLIAM A. BIRD,	WARREN BRYANT,
SHERMAN S. JEWETT,	JOHN ALLEN, Jr.,
C. F. S. THOMAS,	DENNIS BOWEN,
WM. P. LETCHWORTH,	ORLANDO ALLEN,

WILLIAM H. GREENE.

Standing Committees of the Board of Managers.

Finance.—The President, *ex-officio*, Chairman; Messrs. Bird, John Allen, Jr., Jewett.

Library.—Rev. Dr. Chester, Messrs. Greene, Armstrong.

Publications.—Messrs. Thomas, William C. Bryant, Bowen.

Papers and Property.—Messrs. Warren Bryant, Letchworth, Armstrong.

Donations and Collections.—Messrs. Orlando Allen, Jewett, Steele.

Membership.—Messrs. Greene, Armstrong, Bowen.

Standing Committees of the Society.

On the increase of the Library.—Millard Fillmore, Joseph Warren, James O. Putnam.

On the increase of Members.—Samuel M. Welch, Solomon S. Guthrie, Josephus N. Larned.

On Donations and Subscriptions.—Samuel G. Cornell, Rufus L. Howard, James Brayley.

On Statistics.—Merwin S. Hawley, William Fleming, James Sweeny.

On Portraits, Pictures and Photographs.—Laurentius G. Sellstedt, George S. Hazard, Henry G. White.

On Local History.—George V. Brown, Samuel M. Chamberlain, Samuel Smith.

On Indian Reminiscences.—Orsamus H. Marshall, John S. Ganson, Ethan H. Howard.

Resident Members.

Abell, William H.
Alberger, William C.
Allen, John Jr.
Allen, Lewis F.
Allen, Orlando
†Allison, Rev. John
Armstrong, George S.
Austin, Benjamin H.
Austin, Stephen G. (life.)
Babcock, George. R.
Bailey, Gordon
Barnum, George G.
Beals, Edward P.
Bell, David
Bemis, Asaph S.
Bird, William A. (life.)
·Blanchard, Amos A.
Blossom, Thomas
Bogert, Lawrence K. Sr.
Bonney, Zoroaster
Bowen, Daniel
Bowen, Dennis (life.)
Box, Henry W.
Brace, Curtis L.
Brayley, James
Breed, F. W.
Brennan, Barnabas H.
Bristol, Dr. Moses
Brunck, Dr. Francis C.
Brown, George V.
Brown, Robert N.
Brown, Thomas
Bryan, George J.
Bryant, George H.
Bryant, Warren
Bryant, William C.
Buell, Jonathan S.
*Bull, Absalom
Bullymore, Richard
Burwell, Dr. George N.
Burwell, Mrs. M.T.(life.)
Bush, Myron P. (life.)
Butler, Theodore
Cary, Dr. Walter (life.)
Caryl, Benjamin C.
Chamberlain, Samuel M.
Champlin, O. H. P.
Cheesman, William
Chester, Albert T., D.D.
Chester, Anson G.
Clapp, Almon M.
Clark, Cyrus
Clark, Dr. John W.
Clark, Seth
Clark, Thomas (life.)
Clarke, Walter, D.D.
Clinton, George W.
Cochrane, Andrew G. C.
Coit, George Jr. (life.)
Cornell, Samuel G. (life)
Cornwell, Francis E.
Cottle, Octavius O.
Cutler, Abner
Cutter, Ammi W.
Cutting, Harmon S.
Dakin, George
Darrow, Noyes
Dart, Erastus D.
Dart, Joseph Jr.
*Daw, Henry
Dee, William H.
De Forest, Cyrus H.
†Deshler, John G.
Dobbins, David P. (life.)
Dodge, Hampton
Dorr, E. P. (life.)
Dorsheimer, Philip
Dorsheimer, Wm. (life.)
Dudley, Thomas J.
Dutton, Edward H.
Efner, Elijah D.
Emslie, Peter
Enos, Laurens
Ensign, Charles (life.)
Evans, Charles W.
Evans, Edwin T.
Evans, James C.
Eustaphieve, Alex. A.
Fargo, William G. (life.)
Farnham, Thomas
Fillmore, Millard (life.)
Fillmore, Millard P.
Fish, Silas H.
Fisher, J. H.
Fiske, William
Fitch Augustus, B.
*Flagg, Samuel D.
Fleming, William
Flint, Charles G.
Follett, Joseph E.
*Forbush, Eliakim B.
Fosdick, John S.
Francis, Julius E. (life.)
Gallagher, Frank B.
Galligan, William

* Deceased. † Removed.

Ganson, John (life.)
Ganson, John S.
Gardner, John H.
Gardner, Noah H.
Gates, George B.
Gilbert, Edwin
Glenny, William H.
Gorham, George
Granger, Warren
Greene, William H.
Grey, David
Grey, Ernst G.
Gridley, Frederick
*Grosvenor, Seth H.
Guthrie, S. S. (life.)
Hall, Nathan K. (life.)
Hall, William Jr.
†Harvey, Alexander W.
Harvey, Dr. Charles W.
Harvey, Dr. Leon F.
Hathaway, Isaac T.
Hawley, Elias S.
Hawley, M. S. (life.)
Hayes, Dr. George E.
Hazard, Edward E.
Hazard, George S.
Hazard, Morris
Heacock, G. W., D. D.
Heywood, Russel H.
Hibbard, Geo. B. (life.)
Hill, Dr. John D.
Hodge, Benjamin
*Hodge, Philander
Hodge, Velorus
Hodge, William
Holland, Nelson
Hollister, Robert
†Hosmer, Geo. W. D.D.
Howard, Austin A.
Howard, E. H. (life.)
Howard, George (life.)
Howard, Rufus L.
Howcutt, John
Howell, Stephen W.
*Hoyt, James G.
Hudson, John T. (life.)
Humason, Gamaliel
Hurlbert, Edwin
Hutchinson, John M.
Ives, William
Jewett, Elam R.
Jewett, S. S. (life.)
†Johnson, Hiram
Johnson, James M.
Jones, Frederick N.
Jones, George
Jonson, George W.
*Joy, Walter
Kasson, William M.
Kendall, Joshua M.
Ketcham, Alonzo R.
Ketchum, George B.
*Ketchum, Jesse
Ketchum, William
Kingsley, Silas
Kip, Henry
Lacy, John T.
Lansing, Henry L.
Larned, Josephus N.
Laverack, William
Leavitt, James S.
Lee, Cyrus P.
Lee, John R.
Letchworth, William P.
Longstreet, Christopher
Loomis, Charles K.
Loomis, Dr. Horatio N.
Lothrop, Dr. Joshua R.
Lovering, W. Jr. (life.)
Lymburner, H. M.
Marsh, Phineas S.
Marshall, Charles D.
Marshall, O. H. (life.)
Martin, Henry (life.)
Marvin, Eurotus (life.)
Marvin, George L.
Mayhew, Jonathan
Maynard, Robert H.
†Meech, Asa B.
Merrill, George N.
Merrill, Ira
Metzger, George
Miller, James
Miller, Wm. F.
†Millikin, Charles A.
Miner, Dr. Julius F.
Monteath, William
Morse, David R.
Nichols, Asher P. (life.)
*Norton, Charles D.
Otis, Calvin N.
Palmer, Everard
*Palmer, George
Park, Paul
Parker, Jason
Parker, Perry G.
Peck, William B.
*Perkins, Thomas G.
Peter, James F.
†Pitkin, Rev. T. C., D.D.
Plimpton, Luman K.
*Porter, Peter A.
Pratt, Pascal P. (life.)
Pratt, Samuel F. (life.)
Prince, George A.
Prosser, Erastus S. (life.)
Putnam, James O.
Ramsdell, Orrin P.
Ranney, Orville W.
†Rich, Edward S.
Richmond, Alonzo
Richmond, Henry A.
Richmond, Moses M.
†Robinson, Coleman T.
Rochester, Dr. T. F. (life.)
Rockwell, Augustus
Rogers, Henry W. (life.)
Rogers, Sherman S.
Root, Francis H. (life.)
Rounds, George W.
Rumrill, Henry
*Rumsey, Aaron (life.)
Rumsey, B. C. (life.)
Rumsey, D. P. (life.)
Sage, John
Salisbury, Guy H. (life.)
*Sawin, Silas
Sawyer, James D.
Scott, George W.
Scott, William K.
Sellstedt, Laurentius G.
Sexton, Jason
Seymour, Erastus B.
Seymour, Horatio

Shaw, Salmon
Sheldon, James
Shelton, William, D.D.
Shepard, John D. (life.)
Shepard, Sidney
Sheppard, James D.
Sherman, Richard J.
Sherwood, Albert
Sherwood, William C.
Shoecraft, James P.
Shumway, Horatio
Sibley, John C.
Skinner, John B. (life.)
Smith, James M. (life.)
Smith, Samuel
Snow, Dr. Reuben G.
Spaulding, E. G. (life.)
Sprague, Eben C.
Sprague, Noah P.
Steele, Oliver G. (life.)
*Sternberg, Pearl L.
Stevenson, Edward L.
Strong, John C.
Strong, William K.
Sweeney, James
Tanner, Alonzo
Taylor, Martin
Thomas, C. F. S. (life.)
Thomas, Horace G.
Thompson, A. Porter
Tifft, George W. (life.)
Tracy, Francis W.
Tripp, Augustus F.
Trowbridge, Dr. John S.
Tuttle, David N.
Tweedy, William
Utley, Horace
Vail, George O.
Van Vleck, Joseph
Verplanck, Isaac A.
Viele, Henry K.
Vought, John H.
Wadsworth, George
Walker, Henry C.
*Warren, Edward S.
Warren, Joseph
Watson, Stephen V. R.
*Weatherly, John L.
Welch, Samuel M.
*Welch, Thos. C. (life.)
Wells, Chandler J.
*Wells, Richard H.
Wells, William
*Wheeler, Rufus
White, Henry A.
White, Henry G.
White, Isaac D.
White, Dr. J. P. (life.)
Wilgus, Nathaniel
Wilkeson, John
Williams, G. T. (life.)
Williams, Richard
Williams, William
Wood, Francis P.
Woodruff, L. C. (life.)
Worthington, S. K.
Wyckoff, Dr. C. C.
Young, Charles E.
Young, William C.

Corresponding Members.

Allen, Richard L., New York.
Andrews, Prof. E. B., Marietta, O.
Babcock, James F., New Haven, Ct.
Babcock, Marcus L., Batavia, N. Y.
Ballard, Horatio, Homer, N. Y.
Barry, Rev. William, Chicago, Ill.
Barry, Gen. Wm. F., Fort Monroe.
*Beers, Seth P., Litchfield, Ct.
Blake, Freeman M., Fort Erie, C. W.
Boyd, Prof. E. J., Monroe, Mich.
Bradish, Prof. Alvah, Fredonia, N. Y.
Brevoort, J. Carson, Brooklyn, N. Y.
Brown, S. G., Pres. Hamilton College.
Brown, Simon, Concord, Mass.
Bull, Wm. H., Bath, Steuben Co., N. Y.
Burroughs, Lorenzo, Albion, N. Y.
Bush, John T., Clifton, C. W.
Butler, Thomas B., Norwalk, Ct.
Cameron, Hugh, La Crosse, Wis.
Campbell, W. W., Cherry Val., N. Y.
Caulkins, Miss F. M., N. London, Ct.
Chamberlain, Melvin, Boston, Mass.
Cheney, T. A., L.L. D., Havana, N. Y.
Chester, Augustin, Washington, D. C.

Childs, George W., Philadelphia, Pa.
Clark, Joshua V. R., Manlius, N. Y.
Cook, Prof. J.P., Jr.,Cambridge,Mass.
Cooley, Thos. M., Ann Arbor, Mich.
Cornell, Ezra, Ithaca, N. Y.
Cowley, Charles, Lowell, Mass.
Dart, William A., Potsdam, N. Y.
Davies, Henry E., New York.
Dean, George W., Washington, D. C.
De Peyster, Gen. J. W., Tivoli, N. Y.
Diven, A. S., Elmira, N. Y.
Dodd, Edward, Argyle, N. Y.
Doolittle, James R., Racine, Wis.
Doty, Lockwood L., Albany, N. Y.
Drake, Samuel G., Boston, Mass.
Draper, Lyman C., Madison, Wis.
Durrie, Daniel S., Madison, Wis.
Dutcher, Luther L., St. Albans, Vt.
Eliot, W. G., St. Louis, Mo.
Evans, Prof. Ellicott, Clinton, N. Y.
Fellows, J.,Corning,Steuben Co.,N.Y.
Flagler, Thomas T., Lockport, N. Y.
Flint, Dr. Austin, New York.
Follett, Oran, Sandusky, O.
Foote, Elial T., New Haven, Ct.
Force, Gen. M. F., Cincinnati, O.
Foster John, Chicago, Ill.
Fox, Benjamin, Springfield, Ill.
Fox, E. Williams, St. Louis, Mo.
Frank, Augustus, Warsaw, N. Y.
Freeman, Dr. S., Saratoga Springs.
Frothingham, W., Albany, N. Y.
Geddes, George, Camillus, N. Y.
Gilman, D. C., New Haven, Ct.
Goodman, A. T., Jr., Cleveland, O.
Gordon, George Wm., Boston, Mass.
Gould, Prof. B. A., Cambridge, Mass.
Granger, Francis, Canandaigua, N.Y.
Gray, Prof. Asa, L.L. D., Cambridge.
Gray, Dr. John P., Utica, N. Y.
Hall, Rev. E., D.D., Auburn, N. Y.
Hall, S. H. P., Binghamton, N. Y.
Hamilton, Dr. Frank H., New York.
Harwood, Com. A. A., Washington.
Hilgard, J. E., Washington, D. C.
Hoadley, Charles, J., Hartford, Ct.
Hodge, Lorin, Jefferson, O.
Holley, George W., Niagara Falls.
Hollister, Gideon N., Litchfield, Ct.
Horsford, Prof. E. N., Cambridge.
Hosmer, James K., Deerfield, Mass.
Hosmer, William H. C., Avon, N. Y.
Hough, Prof. G. W., Albany, N. Y.
Houghton, George F., St. Albans, Vt.
Huidekoper, Alfred, Meadville, Pa.
Hunt, T. Sterry, L.L. D., Montreal.
Huntington, Edward, Rome, N. Y.
Irvine, William A., Irvine, Pa.
James, John H., Urbana, O.
Jarvis, Edward, Dorchester, Mass.
Jones, Morven M., Utica, N. Y.
Kelley, William, Rhinebeck, N. Y.
Kellogg, A. Otis, M. D., Utica, N. Y.
Kennedy, Joseph C. G., Washington.
King, Charles, L.L. D., New York.
*King, Gov. John A., Jamaica, N.Y.
Kingman, Eliab, Washington, D. C.
Kirtland, Jared P., Cleveland, O.
Kite, Nathan, Philadelphia, Pa.
*Leake, Isaac Q., Jackson, Mich.
Lee, Dr. Charles A., Peekskill, N. Y.
Lewis, Dr. Winslow, Boston, Mass.
Loomis, Prof. E., L.L.D., N. Hav. Ct.
Lewis, George W., Fredonia, N. Y.
Love, John L., San Francisco, Cal.
Lovering, Prof. J., Cambridge, Mass.
Luckey, Rev. Sam'l, Rochester, N.Y.
Lyman, Prof. C. S., New Haven, Ct.
McMaster, Guy H., Bath, N. Y.
Marvin, Richard P., Jamestown, N.Y.
Merritt, J. P., St. Catharines, C. W.
Mix, David E. E., Batavia, N. Y.
Moore, E. M., Rochester, N. Y.
Morgan, Edwin D., New York.
Morgan, Lewis H., Rochester, N. Y.
Moulton, J. W., Roslyn, L. I., N. Y.
Mullen, Joseph, Watertown, N. Y.
Munsell, Joel, Albany, N. Y.
Murphy, Henry C., Brooklyn, N. Y.
Mygatt, Henry R., Oxford, N. Y.
Nason, Rev. E., Billerica Mills, Mass.
Newberry, Prof. J. S., Columbia Col.
Norton, Judge E., San Francisco, Cal.
O'Callaghan, E. B., Albany, N. Y.
O'Reilly, Henry, New York.
Parker, Amasa J., Albany, N. Y.

Parkman, Francis, Boston, Mass.
Peacock, William, Mayville, N. Y.
Pearson, Prof. Jona., Union College.
Perkins, Prof. Geo. R., Utica, N. Y.
Peters, Theodore C., Virginia.
Phelps, Edward J., Burlington, Vt.
Phelps, James A., Titusville, Pa.
Phinney, Elihu, New York.
Plumb, Rev. A. H., Chelsea, Mass.
Pool, Fitch, Danvers, Mass.
Porter, Albert A., Niagara Falls.
Porter, Albert H., Niagara Falls.
Porter, Augustus S., Niagara Falls.
Pratt, Elon G., St. Louis, Mo.
Pratt, Zadock, Prattsville, N. Y.
Pruyn, John V. L., Albany, N. Y.
Randall, H. S., Cortland Village, N. Y.
Redfield, Heman J., Batavia, N. Y.
Reed, Charles M., Erie, Pa.
Safford, Prof. J. M., Nashville, Tenn.
Sandford, Laura G., Erie, Pa.
Saxton, Gen. Rufus, U. S. Army.
Sewall, E. Quincy, Watertown, N. Y.
Shipman, Wm. D., Hartford, Ct.
Silliman, Prof. Benj., New Haven, Ct.
Simpson, Brig. Gen. J. H., Washington.
Sims, Jeptha, Fort Plain, N. Y.
Skinner, J. B. 2d, Attica, N. Y.
Skinner, St. John B. L., Washington.
Smalley, David A., Burlington, Vt.
Smith, George, Upper Darby, N. Y.
*Smith, Junius A., Batavia, N. Y.
Soper, Horace U., Batavia, N. Y.
Spaulding, Lyman A., Lockport, N. Y.
*Spencer, Platt B., Geneva, O.
Stevens, Alden S., Attica, N. Y.
Stone, Wm. L., Saratoga Springs.
Storrs, Wm. C., Rochester, N. Y.
Street, Alfred B., Albany, N. Y.
Strong, Nathaniel T., Irving, N. Y.
Taylor, Col. Rodney M., Washington.
Thompson, Rev. M. L. R. P., Jamest'n.
Tillman, Prof. Samuel D., New York.
Titus, James M., New York.
Trask, Wm. B., Boston, Mass.
Trowbridge, Thos. R., New Haven, Ct.
Trumbull, J. Hammond, Hartford, Ct.
Turner, Nath. A., E. Aurora, Erie Co.
Tyson, Philip R., Baltimore, Md.
Upham, Chas. W., Salem, Mass.
Van Schaak, Henry C., Manlius, N. Y.
Van Tassel, T., Salina, N. Y.
Vinton, Rev. J. A., D.D., Boston, Mass.
*Wadsworth, Gen. J. S., Geneseo, N. Y.
Wadsworth, James, New York.
Waite, John T., Norwich, Ct.
Walker, Edward C., Detroit, Mich.
Walker, Prof. Chas. R., Detroit, Mich.
Walker, Rev. J. B. R., Hartford, Ct.
*Walworth, R. Hyde, Saratoga Spr'gs.
Weed, Monroe, Wyoming, N. Y.
Wells, H., Aurora, Cayuga Co., N. Y.
Wendell, Geo., Mackinac, Mich.
West, Prof. Chas. E., Brooklyn, N. Y.
White, Henry, New Haven, Ct.
Whitehead, A. P., Newark, N. J.
Whiting, William, Boston, Mass.
Whittlesey, Col. C., Cleveland, O.
Wilkeson, Samuel, New York.
Willis, William, Portland, Me.
Wilson, Dr. Peter, Versailles, N. Y.
Winchell, Prof. A., Ann Arbor, Mich.
Woodruff, Maj. Israel C., Washington.
Woolworth, Samuel B., Albany, N. Y.
Worthen, Prof. A. H., Springfield, Ill.
Wright, Rev. A. P., Versailles, N. Y.
Younglove, T. M., Hammondsp't, N. Y.

Honorary Members.

Bancroft, George, New York.
Barnard, F. A. P., Pres. Colum. Col.
Buckingham, Gov. W.A., Norwich, Ct.
*Cass, Lewis, Detroit, Mich.
De Peyster, Frederick, New York.
*Dickinson, D. S., Binghamton, N.Y.
Dix, Gen. John A., New York.
*Everett, Edward, Boston, Mass.
Fisher, Rev. S.W., D.D., Utica, N.Y.
Hall, William, Sr., Cleveland, O.
Hall, Hiland, North Bennington, Vt.
Hawley, Gov. Joseph R., Hartford, Ct.
Hill, Edgar C., Lewiston, N. Y.
Hopkins, Mark, Pres. Williams Col.
Jouett, St. Com. J., Williamst'n, Mass.
Lea, Isaac, L.L.D., Philadelphia, Pa.
Peabody, George, London, England.
Ruggles, Samuel B., New York.
*Scott, Lt. Gen. Winfield, New York.
Storrs, Lucius, Cortland Village, N.Y.
Washburn, Emory, Cambridge, Mass.
Wetherall, Benj. F. H., Detroit, Mich.
Wool, Gen. John E., Troy, N. Y.

INDEX.

www.ingramcontent.com/pod-product-compliance
Lightning Source LLC
LaVergne TN
LVHW011143110826
845150LV00008B/2488

* 9 7 8 1 4 1 8 1 9 1 8 1 8 *